Diffuser Recipes

How to use Aromatherapy and Essential Oils for Better Health, Sleep and Weight Loss

ISBN-13: 978-1973743453
ISBN-10: 1973743450

Table of Contents

Get Our Newest Books For FREE!

We love writing about ways to improve your health.

If you want to receive a FREE COPY of any future books that we release, please sign up to our VIP list.

To show our appreciation, after confirming your subscription, you will be able to download the FREE BONUS report below.

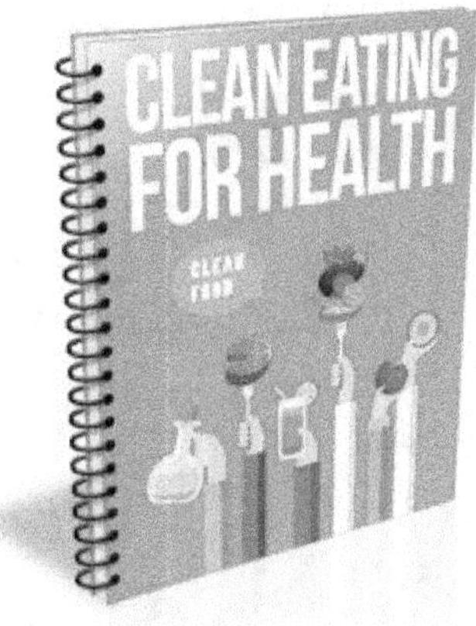

www.restrolla.com/VIP-CoBLo

Introduction

Welcome to *'Diffuser Recipes'*. I hope you find the book informative in your quest to understand how essential oils and combinations of them can help with a variety of health conditions to ensure your wellbeing.

The beauty and wellness industry often markets their products as 'with the goodness of essential oils.' When you go to buy the products you will notice, however, that although they are made from essential oils, they are also laced with other chemical agents which may not be a good solution in the long term. So, what does one do if they want the goodness of essential oils but without having to opt for over the counter products?

The answer is simple – make your own recipes for health, beauty and wellness using essential oils.

For the uninitiated, this book will serve as a *perfect guidebook for essential oil diffuser recipes*, which can be made from the comfort of your home, without denting a hole in your pocket.

It is important to use *highest quality grade essential oils*. These can usually be used both for diffusing, but also for topical (on the skin) application, and sometimes ingested. Therefore, always make sure that you use the best quality oil, and if in doubt, use *'therapeutic grade'* oils, which are labeled safe by the FDA (the Food and Drug Administration in the USA).

To make it easy for you to find your way around the *79 recipes* that I would like to invite you to try, the book is divided into seven chapters, with links from the contents page to 'jump' to the relevant recipe in an instant:

1. Energy

2. Weight loss

3. Sleep disorders

4. Depression & Anxiety

5. Anger

6. Stress

7. Miscellaneous (including recipes to help with allergies, immune function and some aphrodisiacs)

These organic essential oil diffuser recipes are *easy to follow* and are *cost efficient* and will give you the same, if not better, results than store bought beauty products. The recipes are concentrated and pure, and designed to be used with *electronic diffusers* (or candle diffusers). As given the pure oil mixes can be used directly in a *nebulizing* diffuser. To use in an *ultrasonic* device, a little water needs to be added to properly aerosolize the oils. Please carefully read the specific instructions for your device to get the best results.

The recipes can be modified and used in more dilute form with *reed diffusers*. For example, add half of the concentrated recipe given in this book to a ¼ cup of a light oil (e.g. apricot kernel oil or safflower oil) and add 2 tbsp of alcohol (e.g. cheap vodka). The alcohol helps to 'thin out' the oil and allows it to travel up the reeds better.

So, without any further ado, let's get started on your journey to better health!

Chapter 1: Essential Oil Diffuser Recipe Blends for Energy

Citrus Cinnamon

Ingredients:

- 40 drops lemon oil
- 20 drops cinnamon bark oil
- 40 drops lime oil

Method:

1. Add all the oils into a clean, dark bottle. Fasten the cap of the bottle.
1. Shake the bottle well to mix the oils completely.
2. Store the bottle in a dark and cool place.

Usage:

Shake the bottle well before use. Add a few drops of oil into your diffuser. Follow the manufacturer's instructions and use the diffuser as instructed.

Energizing Blends

Ingredients:

- 40 drops rosemary oil
- 60 drops bergamot oil

Method:

1. Add all the oils into a clean, dark bottle. Fasten the cap of the bottle.
2. Shake the bottle well to mix the oils completely.
3. Store the bottle in a dark and cool place.

Usage:

Shake the bottle well before use. Add a few drops of oil into your diffuser. Follow the manufacturer's instructions and use the diffuser.

Beautiful Day Blend

Ingredients:

- 80 drops grapefruit oil
- 20 drops frankincense oil
- 40 drops eucalyptus oil
- 20 drops juniper berry oil

Method:

1. Add all the oils into a clean, dark bottle. Fasten the cap of the bottle.
2. Shake the bottle well to mix the oils completely.
3. Store the bottle in a dark and cool place.

Usage:

Shake the bottle well before use. Add a few drops of oil into your diffuser. Follow the manufacturer's instructions and use the diffuser as instructed.

Instant Energy

Ingredients:

- 40 drops peppermint oil
- 20 drops lime oil
- 40 drops orange oil

Method:

1. Add all the oils into a clean, dark bottle. Fasten the cap of the bottle.
2. Shake the bottle well to mix the oils completely.
3. Store the bottle in a dark and cool place.

Usage:

Shake the bottle well before use. Add a few drops of oil into your diffuser. Follow the manufacturer's instructions and use the diffuser as instructed.

Fatigue Fighter

Ingredients:

- 60 drops bergamot oil
- 20 drops peppermint oil
- 40 drops grapefruit oil

Method:

1. Add all the oils into a clean, dark bottle. Fasten the cap of the bottle.
2. Shake the bottle well to mix the oils completely.
3. Store the bottle in a dark and cool place.

Usage:

Shake the bottle well before use. Add a few drops of oil into your diffuser. Follow the manufacturer's instructions and use the diffuser as instructed.

Chapter 2: Essential Oil Diffuser Recipe Blends for Weight Loss

Appetite Suppressing Diffusion

Ingredients:

- 25 drops ginger oil
- 40 drops lemon oil
- 80 drops mandarin oil
- 25 drops peppermint oil

Method:

1. Add all the oils into a clean, dark bottle. Fasten the cap of the bottle.
2. Shake the bottle well to mix the oils completely.
3. Store the bottle in a dark and cool place.

Usage:

Shake the bottle well before use. Add a few drops of oil into your diffuser. Follow the manufacturer's instructions and use the diffuser as instructed.

Cinnamon and Lime Blend

Ingredients:

- 20 drops grapefruit oil
- 20 drops lime oil
- 20 drops peppermint oil
- 20 drops cinnamon oil

Method:

1. Add all the oils into a clean, dark bottle. Fasten the cap of the bottle.
2. Shake the bottle well to mix the oils completely.
3. Store the bottle in a dark and cool place.

Usage:

Shake the bottle well before use. Add a few drops of oil into your diffuser. Follow the manufacturer's instructions and use the diffuser as instructed.

Citrus Weight Loss Blend

Ingredients:

- 60 drops grapefruit oil
- 2 drops ylang ylang oil
- 8 drops lemon oil

Method:

1. Add all the oils into a clean, dark bottle. Fasten the cap of the bottle.
2. Shake the bottle well to mix the oils completely.
3. Store the bottle in a dark and cool place.

Usage:

Shake the bottle well before use. Add a few drops of oil into your diffuser. Follow the manufacturer's instructions and use the diffuser as instructed.

Mint Weight Loss Blend

Ingredients:

- 40 drops peppermint oil
- 8 drops spearmint oil
- 20 drops bergamot oil
- 2 drops ylang ylang oil

Method:

1. Add all the oils into a clean, dark bottle. Fasten the cap of the bottle.
2. Shake the bottle well to mix the oils completely.
3. Store the bottle in a dark and cool place.

Usage:

Shake the bottle well before use. Add a few drops of oil into your diffuser. Follow the manufacturer's instructions and use the diffuser as instructed.

Herbal Weight Loss Blend

Ingredients:

- 30 drops marjoram oil
- 30 drops basil oil
- 2 drops thyme oil
- 2 drops oregano oil

Method:

1. Add all the oils into a clean, dark bottle. Fasten the cap of the bottle.
2. Shake the bottle well to mix the oils completely.
3. Store the bottle in a dark and cool place.

Usage:

Shake the bottle well before use. Add a few drops of oil into your diffuser. Follow the manufacturer's instructions and use the diffuser as instructed.

'No Thanks, I am full' Diffuser blend

Ingredients:

- 30 drops lemon oil
- 30 drops grapefruit oil
- 10 drops ylang ylang oil
- 10 drops spearmint oil

Method:

1. Add all the oils into a clean, dark bottle. Fasten the cap of the bottle.
2. Shake the bottle well to mix the oils completely.
3. Store the bottle in a dark and cool place.

Usage:

Shake the bottle well before use. Add a few drops of oil into your diffuser. Follow the manufacturer's instructions and use the diffuser as instructed.

Chapter 3: Essential Oil Diffuser Recipe Blends for Sleep Disorders

Good Night Sleep Tight Blend

Ingredients:

- 35 drops lavender oil
- 15 drops Roman chamomile oil
- 22 drops sweet marjoram oil
- 15 drops bergamot oil
- 3 drops valerian root oil
- 3 drops ylang ylang oil

Method:

1. Add all the oils into a clean, dark bottle. Fasten the cap of the bottle.
2. Shake the bottle well to mix the oils completely.
3. Store the bottle in a dark and cool place.

Usage:

Shake the bottle well before use. Add a few drops of oil into your diffuser. Follow the manufacturer's instructions and use the diffuser as instructed. Use the diffuser a few minutes before bedtime.

Sleeptime #1

Ingredients:

- 20 drops marjoram oil
- 20 drops lavender oil
- 20 drops slim and sassy oil

Method:

1. Add all the oils into a clean, dark bottle. Fasten the cap of the bottle.
2. Shake the bottle well to mix the oils completely.
3. Store the bottle in a dark and cool place.

Usage:

Shake the bottle well before use. Add a few drops of oil into your diffuser. Follow the manufacturer's instructions and use the diffuser as instructed. Use the diffuser a few minutes before bedtime.

Sleeptime #2

Ingredients:

- 30drops wild orange oil
- 30 drops serenity oil

Method:

1. Add all the oils into a clean, dark bottle. Fasten the cap of the bottle.
2. Shake the bottle well to mix the oils completely.
3. Store the bottle in a dark and cool place.

Usage:

Shake the bottle well before use. Add a few drops of oil into your diffuser. Follow the manufacturer's instructions and use the diffuser as instructed. Use the diffuser a few minutes before bedtime.

Sleeptime #3

Ingredients:

- 20 drops lavender oil
- 20 drops wild orange oil
- 20 drops cedar wood oil

Method:

1. Add all the oils into a clean, dark bottle. Fasten the cap of the bottle.
2. Shake the bottle well to mix the oils completely.
3. Store the bottle in a dark and cool place.

Usage:

Shake the bottle well before use. Add a few drops of oil into your diffuser. Follow the manufacturer's instructions and use the diffuser as instructed. Use the diffuser a few minutes before bedtime.

Sleeptime #4

Ingredients:

- 20 drops wild orange oil
- 40 drops peace oil

Method:

1. Add all the oils into a clean, dark bottle. Fasten the cap of the bottle.
2. Shake the bottle well to mix the oils completely.
3. Store the bottle in a dark and cool place.

Usage:

Shake the bottle well before use. Add a few drops of oil into your diffuser. Follow the manufacturer's instructions and use the diffuser as instructed. Use the diffuser a few minutes before bedtime.

Sleeptime #5

Ingredients:

- 20 drops vetiver oil
- 30 drops bergamot oil
- 10 drops sandalwood oil

Method:

1. Add all the oils into a clean, dark bottle. Fasten the cap of the bottle.
2. Shake the bottle well to mix the oils completely.
3. Store the bottle in a dark and cool place.

Usage:

Shake the bottle well before use. Add a few drops of oil into your diffuser. Follow the manufacturer's instructions and use the diffuser as instructed. Use the diffuser a few minutes before bedtime.

Sleeptime #6

Ingredients:

- 30 drops Roman chamomile oil
- 30 drops lavender oil
- 20 drops ylang ylang oil

Method:

1. Add all the oils into a clean, dark bottle. Fasten the cap of the bottle.
2. Shake the bottle well to mix the oils completely.
3. Store the bottle in a dark and cool place.

Usage:

Shake the bottle well before use. Add a few drops of oil into your diffuser. Follow the manufacturer's instructions and use the diffuser as instructed. Use the diffuser a few minutes before bedtime.

"Make Me Sleepy" Diffuser for Sleep

Ingredients:

- 20 drops Roman chamomile oil
- 10 drops bergamot oil
- 10 drops Clary sage oil

Method:

1. Add all the oils into a clean, dark dropper bottle. Fasten the cap of the bottle.
2. Shake the bottle well to mix the oils completely.
3. Store the bottle in a dark and cool place.

Usage:

Shake the bottle well before use. Add a few drops of oil into your diffuser. Follow the manufacturer's instructions and use the diffuser as instructed. Use the diffuser a few minutes before bedtime.

"Restful Slumber"

Ingredients:

- 40 drops lavender oil
- 20 drops neroli oil
- 20 drops cedar wood oil

Method:

1. Add all the oils into a clean, dark dropper bottle. Fasten the cap of the bottle.
2. Shake the bottle well to mix the oils completely.
3. Store the bottle in a dark and cool place.

Usage:

Shake the bottle well before use. Add a few drops of oil into your diffuser. Follow the manufacturer's instructions and use the diffuser as instructed. Use the diffuser a few minutes before bedtime.

"Calm Me Down" Sleep Aid

Ingredients:

- 40 drops frankincense oil
- 20 drops wild orange oil
- 20 drops rosemary oil

Method:

1. Add all the oils into a clean, dark dropper bottle. Fasten the cap of the bottle.
2. Shake the bottle well to mix the oils completely.
3. Store the bottle in a dark and cool place.

Usage:

Shake the bottle well before use. Add a few drops of oil into your diffuser. Follow the manufacturer's instructions and use the diffuser as instructed. Use the diffuser a few minutes before bedtime.

Sleep Aid for Snoring

Ingredients:

- 40 drops geranium oil
- 40 drops lavender oil
- 40 drops marjoram oil
- 16 drops eucalyptus oil
- 16 drops cedar wood oil
- 8 drops frankincense oil

Method:

1. Add all the oils into a clean, dark dropper bottle. Fasten the cap of the bottle.
2. Shake the bottle well to mix the oils completely.
3. Store the bottle in a dark and cool place.

Usage:

Shake the bottle well before use. Add a few drops of oil into your diffuser. Follow the manufacturer's instructions and use the diffuser as instructed. Use the diffuser a few minutes before bedtime.

This blend is also good for those who have blocked nasal passages, allergies etc.

Blend for Snoring

Ingredients:

- 20 drops lavender oil
- 20 drops tea tree oil

Method:

1. Add all the oils into a clean, dark dropper bottle. Fasten the cap of the bottle.
2. Shake the bottle well to mix the oils completely.
3. Store the bottle in a dark and cool place.

Usage:

Shake the bottle well before use. Add a few drops of oil into your diffuser. Follow the manufacturer's instructions and use the diffuser as instructed.

You can also use only lavender oil or only tea tree oil to combat snoring.

Sleep Aid for Sleep Apnea

Ingredients:

- 15 drops peppermint oil
- 25 drops lavender oil

Method:

1. Add all the oils into a clean, dark dropper bottle. Fasten the cap of the bottle.
2. Shake the bottle well to mix the oils completely.
3. Store the bottle in a dark and cool place.

Usage:

Shake the bottle well before use. Add a few drops of oil into your diffuser. Follow the manufacturer's instructions and use the diffuser as instructed. Use the diffuser a few minutes before bedtime.

Essential Oil Blend for Sleep Walking

Ingredients:

- 20 drops frankincense oil
- 20 drops blue tansy oil
- 20 drops spruce oil
- 20 drops rosewood oil

Method:

1. Add all the oils into a clean, dark dropper bottle. Fasten the cap of the bottle.
2. Shake the bottle well to mix the oils completely.
3. Store the bottle in a dark and cool place.

Usage:

Shake the bottle well before use. Add a few drops of oil into your diffuser. Follow the manufacturer's instructions and use the diffuser as instructed. Use the diffuser a few minutes before bedtime.

Chapter 4: Essential Oil Diffuser Recipe Blends for Depression

Anti-depressant Blend #1

Ingredients:

- 40 drops bergamot oil
- 20 drops vetiver oil
- 20 drops Clary sage oil

Method:

1. Add all the oils into a clean, dark dropper bottle. Fasten the cap of the bottle.
2. Shake the bottle well to mix the oils completely.
3. Store the bottle in a dark and cool place.

Usage:

Shake the bottle well before use. Add about 20 drops of the oil blend into about 1/3 cup water to use in your diffuser. Follow the manufacturer's instructions and use the diffuser as instructed.

Anti-depressant Blend #2

Ingredients:

- 20 drops lavender oil
- 40 drops neroli oil
- 20 drops sandal wood oil
- 40 drops ylang ylang oil

Method:

1. Add all the oils into a clean, dark dropper bottle. Fasten the cap of the bottle.
2. Shake the bottle well to mix the oils completely.
3. Store the bottle in a dark and cool place.

Usage:

Shake the bottle well before use. Add about 20 drops of the oil blend into about 1/3 cup water to use in your diffuser. Follow the manufacturer's instructions and use the diffuser as instructed.

Anti-anxiety Blend

Ingredients:

- 32 drops sandalwood oil
- 16 drops rose oil
- 16 drops bergamot oil
- 8 drops orange oil

Method:

1. Add all the oils into a clean, dark dropper bottle. Fasten the cap of the bottle.
2. Shake the bottle well to mix the oils completely.
3. Store the bottle in a dark and cool place.

Usage:

Shake the bottle well before use. Add a few drops of oil into your diffuser. Follow the manufacturer's instructions and use the diffuser as instructed.

Anxious Depression Blend

Ingredients:

- 32 drops grapefruit oil
- 32 drops lavender oil
- 8 drops marjoram oil
- 4 drops geranium oil
- 4 drops Roman chamomile oil

Method:

1. Add all the oils into a clean, dark dropper bottle. Fasten the cap of the bottle.
2. Shake the bottle well to mix the oils completely.
3. Store the bottle in a dark and cool place.

Usage:

Shake the bottle well before use. Add a few drops of oil into your diffuser. Follow the manufacturer's instructions and use the diffuser as instructed.

Mood Lifter

Ingredients:

- 40 drops bergamot oil
- 16 drops wild orange oil
- 20 drops grapefruit oil
- 4 drops geranium oil
- 4 drops ylang ylang oil

Method:

1. Add all the oils into a clean, dark dropper bottle. Fasten the cap of the bottle.
2. Shake the bottle well to mix the oils completely.
3. Store the bottle in a dark and cool place.

Usage:

Shake the bottle well before use. Add a few drops of oil into your diffuser. Follow the manufacturer's instructions and use the diffuser as instructed.

Simple Depression Relief Blend

Ingredients:

- 40 drops Clary sage oil
- 10 drops sandalwood oil
- 20 drops basil oil
- 30 drops geranium oil
- 40 drops ylang ylang oil

Method:

1. Add all the oils into a clean, dark dropper bottle. Fasten the cap of the bottle.
2. Shake the bottle well to mix the oils completely.
3. Store the bottle in a dark and cool place.

Usage:

Shake the bottle well before use. Add a few drops of oil into your diffuser. Follow the manufacturer's instructions and use the diffuser as instructed.

Anti-depression and Anti-Anxiety Blend #1

Ingredients:

- 30 drops sandalwood oil
- 10 drops rose oil
- 10 drops orange oil

Method:

1. Add all the oils into a clean, dark dropper bottle. Fasten the cap of the bottle.
2. Shake the bottle well to mix the oils completely.
3. Store the bottle in a dark and cool place.

Usage:

Shake the bottle well before use. Add a few drops of oil into your diffuser. Follow the manufacturer's instructions and use the diffuser as instructed.

Anti-Depression and Anti-Anxiety Blend #2

Ingredients:

- 40 drops Clary sage oil
- 60 drops bergamot oil

Method:

1. Add all the oils into a clean, dark dropper bottle. Fasten the cap of the bottle.
2. Shake the bottle well to mix the oils completely.
3. Store the bottle in a dark and cool place.

Usage:

Shake the bottle well before use. Add a few drops of oil into your diffuser. Follow the manufacturer's instructions and use the diffuser as instructed.

This blend is also helps in overcoming loneliness.

Anti-Depression and Anti-Anxiety Blend #3

Ingredients:

- 30 drops grapefruit oil
- 10 drops ylang ylang oil
- 10 drops lavender

Method:

1. Add all the oils into a clean, dark dropper bottle. Fasten the cap of the bottle.
2. Shake the bottle well to mix the oils completely.
3. Store the bottle in a dark and cool place.

Usage:

Shake the bottle well before use. Add a few drops of oil into your diffuser. Follow the manufacturer's instructions and use the diffuser as instructed.

Anti-Depression and Anti-Anxiety Blend #4

Ingredients:

- 40 drops frankincense oil
- 20 drops jasmine oil or neroli oil
- 10 drops lemon oil

Method:

1. Add all the oils into a clean, dark dropper bottle. Fasten the cap of the bottle.
2. Shake the bottle well to mix the oils completely.
3. Store the bottle in a dark and cool place.

Usage:

Shake the bottle well before use. Add a few drops of oil into your diffuser. Follow the manufacturer's instructions and use the diffuser as instructed.

Mood Lifter for Irritable Depression

Ingredients:

- 40 drops bergamot oil
- 16 drops sweet orange oil
- 20 drops grapefruit oil
- 10 drops ylang ylang oil
- 10 drops geranium oil

Method:

1. Add all the oils into a clean, dark dropper bottle. Fasten the cap of the bottle.
2. Shake the bottle well to mix the oils completely.
3. Store the bottle in a dark and cool place.

Usage:

Shake the bottle well before use. Add a few drops of oil into your diffuser. Follow the manufacturer's instructions and use the diffuser as instructed.

Comforting Blend for Grief Related Depression

Ingredients:

- 40 drops rose absolute or rose Otto oil
- 16 drops Petitgrain or neroli oil
- 16 drops sandalwood oil

Method:

1. Add all the oils into a clean, dark dropper bottle. Fasten the cap of the bottle.
2. Shake the bottle well to mix the oils completely.
3. Store the bottle in a dark and cool place.

Usage:

Shake the bottle well before use. Add a few drops of oil into your diffuser. Follow the manufacturer's instructions and use the diffuser as instructed.

Soothing Blend for Anxious Depression

Ingredients:

- 32 drops grapefruit oil
- 8 drops marjoram oil
- 32 drops lavender oil
- 2 drops chamomile oil
- 2 drops geranium oil

Method:

1. Add all the oils into a clean, dark dropper bottle. Fasten the cap of the bottle.
2. Shake the bottle well to mix the oils completely.
3. Store the bottle in a dark and cool place.

Usage:

Shake the bottle well before use. Add a few drops of oil into your diffuser. Follow the manufacturer's instructions and use the diffuser as instructed.

Anxiety Blend #1

Ingredients:

- 5 drops Roman chamomile oil
- 25 drops sandalwood oil
- 5 drops neroli oil
- 5 drops lavender oil

Method:

1. Add all the oils into a clean, dark dropper bottle. Fasten the cap of the bottle.
2. Shake the bottle well to mix the oils completely.
3. Store the bottle in a dark and cool place.

Usage:

Shake the bottle well before use. Add a few drops of oil into your diffuser. Follow the manufacturer's instructions and use the diffuser as instructed.

Anxiety Blend #2

Ingredients:

- 40 drops bergamot oil
- 20 drops frankincense oil
- 40 drops Clary sage oil

Method:

1. Add all the oils into a clean, dark dropper bottle. Fasten the cap of the bottle.
2. Shake the bottle well to mix the oils completely.
3. Store the bottle in a dark and cool place.

Usage:

Shake the bottle well before use. Add a few drops of oil into your diffuser. Follow the manufacturer's instructions and use the diffuser as instructed.

Anxiety Blend #3

Ingredients:

- 40 drops bergamot oil
- 60 drops sandalwood oil

Method:

1. Add all the oils into a clean, dark dropper bottle. Fasten the cap of the bottle.
2. Shake the bottle well to mix the oils completely.
3. Store the bottle in a dark and cool place.

Usage:

Shake the bottle well before use. Add a few drops of oil into your diffuser. Follow the manufacturer's instructions and use the diffuser as instructed.

Anxiety Blend #4

Ingredients:

- 30 drops Clary sage oil
- 45 drops lavender oil

Method:

1. Add all the oils into a clean, dark dropper bottle. Fasten the cap of the bottle.
2. Shake the bottle well to mix the oils completely.
3. Store the bottle in a dark and cool place.

Usage:

Shake the bottle well before use. Add a few drops of oil into your diffuser. Follow the manufacturer's instructions and use the diffuser as instructed.

Anxiety Blend #5

Ingredients:

- 20 drops rose oil
- 40 drops mandarin oil
- 20 drops lavender oil
- 10 drops vetiver oil

Method:

1. Add all the oils into a clean, dark dropper bottle. Fasten the cap of the bottle.
2. Shake the bottle well to mix the oils completely.
3. Store the bottle in a dark and cool place.

Usage:

Shake the bottle well before use. Add a few drops of oil into your diffuser. Follow the manufacturer's instructions and use the diffuser as instructed.

Chapter 5: Essential Oil Diffuser Recipe Blends for Anger

Anti-anger Blend #1

Ingredients:

- 30 drops orange oil
- 10 drops rose oil
- 10 drops vetiver

Method:

1. Add all the oils into a clean, dark dropper bottle. Fasten the cap of the bottle.
2. Shake the bottle well to mix the oils completely.
3. Store the bottle in a dark and cool place.

Usage:

Shake the bottle well before use. Add a few drops of oil into your diffuser. Follow the manufacturer's instructions and use the diffuser as instructed.

Anti-anger Blend #2

Ingredients:

- 30 drops bergamot oil
- 10 drops jasmine oil
- 10 drops ylang ylang oil

Method:

1. Add all the oils into a clean, dark dropper bottle. Fasten the cap of the bottle.
2. Shake the bottle well to mix the oils completely.
3. Store the bottle in a dark and cool place.

Usage:

Shake the bottle well before use. Add a few drops of oil into your diffuser. Follow the manufacturer's instructions and use the diffuser as instructed.

Anti-anger Blend #3

Ingredients:

- 20 drops orange oil
- 20 drops bergamot oil
- 10 drops Roman chamomile oil

Method:

1. Add all the oils into a clean, dark dropper bottle. Fasten the cap of the bottle.
2. Shake the bottle well to mix the oils completely.
3. Store the bottle in a dark and cool place.

Usage:

Shake the bottle well before use. Add a few drops of oil into your diffuser. Follow the manufacturer's instructions and use the diffuser as instructed.

Anti-anger Blend #4

Ingredients:

- 40 drops patchouli oil
- 60 drops orange oil

Method:

1. Add all the oils into a clean, dark dropper bottle. Fasten the cap of the bottle.
2. Shake the bottle well to mix the oils completely.
3. Store the bottle in a dark and cool place.

Usage:

Shake the bottle well before use. Add a few drops of oil into your diffuser. Follow the manufacturer's instructions and use the diffuser as instructed.

Chapter 6: Essential Oil Diffuser Recipe Blends for Stress

Anti-stress Blend #1

Ingredients:

- 20 drops lavender oil
- 10 drops orange oil
- 30 drops frankincense oil

Method:

1. Add all the oils into a clean, dark dropper bottle. Fasten the cap of the bottle.
2. Shake the bottle well to mix the oils completely.
3. Store the bottle in a dark and cool place.

Usage:

Shake the bottle well before use. Add a few drops of oil into your diffuser. Follow the manufacturer's instructions and use the diffuser as instructed.

Anti-stress Blend #2

Ingredients:

- 30 drops lavender oil
- 30 drops Roman chamomile oil
- 20 drops ylang ylang oil

Method:

1. Add all the oils into a clean, dark dropper bottle. Fasten the cap of the bottle.
2. Shake the bottle well to mix the oils completely.
3. Store the bottle in a dark and cool place.

Usage:

Shake the bottle well before use. Add a few drops of oil into your diffuser. Follow the manufacturer's instructions and use the diffuser as instructed.

Anti-stress Blend #3

Ingredients:

- 40 drops lavender oil
- 20 drops mandarin oil
- 20 drops lime oil

Method:

1. Add all the oils into a clean, dark dropper bottle. Fasten the cap of the bottle.
2. Shake the bottle well to mix the oils completely.
3. Store the bottle in a dark and cool place.

Usage:

Shake the bottle well before use. Add a few drops of oil into your diffuser. Follow the manufacturer's instructions and use the diffuser as instructed.

Anti-stress Blend #4

Ingredients:

- 40 drops lavender oil
- 40 drops bergamot oil
- 20 drops geranium oil

Method:

1. Add all the oils into a clean, dark dropper bottle. Fasten the cap of the bottle.
2. Shake the bottle well to mix the oils completely.
3. Store the bottle in a dark and cool place.

Usage:

Shake the bottle well before use. Add a few drops of oil into your diffuser. Follow the manufacturer's instructions and use the diffuser as instructed.

Anti-stress Blend #5

Ingredients:

- 30 drops lavender oil
- 30 drops lemon oil
- 90 drops Clary sage oil

Method:

1. Add all the oils into a clean, dark dropper bottle. Fasten the cap of the bottle.
2. Shake the bottle well to mix the oils completely.
3. Store the bottle in a dark and cool place.

Usage:

Shake the bottle well before use. Add a few drops of oil into your diffuser. Follow the manufacturer's instructions and use the diffuser as instructed.

Anti-stress Blend #6

Ingredients:

- 50 drops lavender oil
- 50 drops Roman chamomile oil
- 25 drops vetiver oil

Method:

1. Add all the oils into a clean, dark dropper bottle. Fasten the cap of the bottle.
2. Shake the bottle well to mix the oils completely.
3. Store the bottle in a dark and cool place.

Usage:

Shake the bottle well before use. Add a few drops of oil into your diffuser. Follow the manufacturer's instructions and use the diffuser as instructed.

Anti-stress Blend #7

Ingredients:

- 75 drops bergamot oil
- 25 drops geranium oil
- 25 drops frankincense oil

Method:

1. Add all the oils into a clean, dark dropper bottle. Fasten the cap of the bottle.
2. Shake the bottle well to mix the oils completely.
3. Store the bottle in a dark and cool place.

Usage:

Shake the bottle well before use. Add a few drops of oil into your diffuser. Follow the manufacturer's instructions and use the diffuser as instructed.

Anti-stress Blend #8

Ingredients:

- 75 drops grapefruit oil
- 25 drops ylang ylang oil
- 25 drops jasmine oil

Method:

1. Add all the oils into a clean, dark dropper bottle. Fasten the cap of the bottle.
2. Shake the bottle well to mix the oils completely.
3. Store the bottle in a dark and cool place.

Usage:

Shake the bottle well before use. Add a few drops of oil into your diffuser. Follow the manufacturer's instructions and use the diffuser as instructed.

Anti-stress Blend #9

Ingredients:

- 30 drops lavender oil
- 30 drops cedar wood oil

Method:

1. Add all the oils into a clean, dark dropper bottle. Fasten the cap of the bottle.
2. Shake the bottle well to mix the oils completely.
3. Store the bottle in a dark and cool place.

Usage:

Shake the bottle well before use. Add a few drops of oil into your diffuser. Follow the manufacturer's instructions and use the diffuser as instructed.

Anti-stress Blend #8

Ingredients:

- 20 drops cedar wood oil
- 10 drops rosemary oil
- 20 drops orange oil
- 20 drops frankincense oil

Method:

1. Add all the oils into a clean, dark dropper bottle. Fasten the cap of the bottle.
2. Shake the bottle well to mix the oils completely.
3. Store the bottle in a dark and cool place.

Usage:

Shake the bottle well before use. Add a few drops of oil into your diffuser. Follow the manufacturer's instructions and use the diffuser as instructed.

Anti-stress Blend #9

Ingredients:

- 30 drops vetiver oil
- 30 drops lavender oil

Method:

1. Add all the oils into a clean, dark dropper bottle. Fasten the cap of the bottle.
2. Shake the bottle well to mix the oils completely.
3. Store the bottle in a dark and cool place.

Usage:

Shake the bottle well before use. Add a few drops of oil into your diffuser. Follow the manufacturer's instructions and use the diffuser as instructed.

Anti-stress Blend #10

Ingredients:

- 30 drops spearmint oil
- 30 drops eucalyptus oil

Method:

1. Add all the oils into a clean, dark dropper bottle. Fasten the cap of the bottle.
2. Shake the bottle well to mix the oils completely.
3. Store the bottle in a dark and cool place.

Usage:

Shake the bottle well before use. Add a few drops of oil into your diffuser. Follow the manufacturer's instructions and use the diffuser as instructed.

Anti-stress Blend #11

Ingredients:

- 20 drops cedar wood oil
- 60 drops lavender oil
- 20 drops ylang ylang oil
- 20 drops wild orange oil

Method:

1. Add all the oils into a clean, dark dropper bottle. Fasten the cap of the bottle.
2. Shake the bottle well to mix the oils completely.
3. Store the bottle in a dark and cool place.

Usage:

Shake the bottle well before use. Add a few drops of oil into your diffuser. Follow the manufacturer's instructions and use the diffuser as instructed.

Anti-stress Blend #12

Ingredients:

- 20 drops patchouli oil
- 20 drops bergamot oil
- 20 drops cypress oil

Method:

1. Add all the oils into a clean, dark dropper bottle. Fasten the cap of the bottle.
2. Shake the bottle well to mix the oils completely.
3. Store the bottle in a dark and cool place.

Usage:

Shake the bottle well before use. Add a few drops of oil into your diffuser. Follow the manufacturer's instructions and use the diffuser as instructed.

"Refresh" Calming Blend

Ingredients:

- 40 drops grapefruit oil
- 40 drops lime oil
- 40 drops bergamot oil
- 40 drops sandalwood oil

Method:

1. Add all the oils into a clean, dark dropper bottle. Fasten the cap of the bottle.
2. Shake the bottle well to mix the oils completely.
3. Store the bottle in a dark and cool place.

Usage:

Shake the bottle well before use. Add a few drops of oil into your diffuser. Follow the manufacturer's instructions and use the diffuser as instructed.

"Stress Less" Calming Blend

Ingredients:

- 30 drops lavender oil
- 10 drops ylang ylang oil
- 20 drops Clary sage oil
- 10 drops marjoram oil

Method:

1. Add all the oils into a clean, dark dropper bottle. Fasten the cap of the bottle.
2. Shake the bottle well to mix the oils completely.
3. Store the bottle in a dark and cool place.

Usage:

Shake the bottle well before use. Add a few drops of oil into your diffuser. Follow the manufacturer's instructions and use the diffuser as instructed.

Stress Management Blend

Ingredients:

- 40 drops cedar wood oil
- 20 drops jasmine oil
- 30 drops bergamot oil
- 10 drops neroli oil

Method:

1. Add all the oils into a clean, dark dropper bottle. Fasten the cap of the bottle.
2. Shake the bottle well to mix the oils completely.
3. Store the bottle in a dark and cool place.

Usage:

Shake the bottle well before use. Add a few drops of oil into your diffuser. Follow the manufacturer's instructions and use the diffuser as instructed.

Stress Away Blend

Ingredients:

- 40 drops lavender oil
- 20 drops ylang ylang oil
- 30 drops Clary sage oil
- 10 drops marjoram oil

Method:

1. Add all the oils into a clean, dark dropper bottle. Fasten the cap of the bottle.
2. Shake the bottle well to mix the oils completely.
3. Store the bottle in a dark and cool place.

Usage:

Shake the bottle well before use. Add a few drops of oil into your diffuser. Follow the manufacturer's instructions and use the diffuser as instructed.

Chapter 7: Essential Oil Diffuser Miscellaneous Recipe Blends

Sensual Blend

Ingredients:

- 25 drops sandalwood oil
- 5 drops ginger oil
- 5 drops ylang ylang oil
- 5 drops lime oil
- 15 drops bergamot oil

Method:

1. Add all the oils into a clean, dark dropper bottle. Fasten the cap of the bottle.
2. Shake the bottle well to mix the oils completely.
3. Store the bottle in a dark and cool place.

Usage:

Shake the bottle well before use. Add a few drops of oil into your diffuser. Follow the manufacturer's instructions and use the diffuser as instructed.

Aphrodisiac Blend

Ingredients:

- 20 drops cinnamon oil
- 10 drops rosemary oil
- 20 drops patchouli oil
- 10 drops ylang ylang oil
- 10 drops sandalwood oil

Method:

1. Add all the oils into a clean, dark dropper bottle. Fasten the cap of the bottle.
2. Shake the bottle well to mix the oils completely.
3. Store the bottle in a dark and cool place.

Usage:

Shake the bottle well before use. Add a few drops of oil into your diffuser. Follow the manufacturer's instructions and use the diffuser as instructed.

Sexy Time Blend

Ingredients:

- 30 drops ylang ylang oil
- 30 drops Idaho blue spruce oil
- 20 drops orange oil
- 20 drops bergamot oil

Method:

1. Add all the oils into a clean, dark dropper bottle. Fasten the cap of the bottle.
2. Shake the bottle well to mix the oils completely.
3. Store the bottle in a dark and cool place.

Usage:

Shake the bottle well before use. Add a few drops of oil into your diffuser. Follow the manufacturer's instructions and use the diffuser as instructed.

Seasonal Discomfort Blend

Ingredients:

- 30 drops lavender oil
- 30 drops lemon oil
- 30 drops peppermint oil

Method:

1. Add all the oils into a clean, dark dropper bottle. Fasten the cap of the bottle.
2. Shake the bottle well to mix the oils completely.
3. Store the bottle in a dark and cool place.

Usage:

Shake the bottle well before use. Add a few drops of oil into your diffuser. Follow the manufacturer's instructions and use the diffuser as instructed.

Headache Blend #1

Ingredients:

- 20 drops marjoram oil
- 20 drops rosemary oil
- 20 drops lavender oil
- 20 drops thyme oil

Method:

1. Add all the oils into a clean, dark dropper bottle. Fasten the cap of the bottle.
2. Shake the bottle well to mix the oils completely.
3. Store the bottle in a dark and cool place.

Usage:

Shake the bottle well before use. Add a few drops of oil into your diffuser. Follow the manufacturer's instructions and use the diffuser as instructed.

Headache Blend #2 for Sinus

Ingredients:

- 45 drops rosemary oil
- 20 drops geranium oil
- 10 drops eucalyptus oil
- 25 drops Melaleuca oil
- 15 drops peppermint oil
- 10 drops lavender oil

Method:

1. Add all the oils into a clean, dark dropper bottle. Fasten the cap of the bottle.
2. Shake the bottle well to mix the oils completely.
3. Store the bottle in a dark and cool place.

Usage:

Shake the bottle well before use. Add a few drops of oil into your diffuser. Follow the manufacturer's instructions and use the diffuser as instructed.

Immune Booster Blend #1

Ingredients:

- 20 drops on guard oil
- 10 drops oregano oil
- 15 drops lemon oil

Method:

1. Add all the oils into a clean, dark dropper bottle. Fasten the cap of the bottle.
2. Shake the bottle well to mix the oils completely.
3. Store the bottle in a dark and cool place.

Usage:

Shake the bottle well before use. Add a few drops of oil into your diffuser. Follow the manufacturer's instructions and use the diffuser as instructed.

Immune Booster Blend #2

Ingredients:

- 10 drops rosemary oil
- 10 drops eucalyptus oil
- 10 drops wild orange oil
- 10 drops clove oil
- 10 drops cinnamon oil

Method:

1. Add all the oils into a clean, dark dropper bottle. Fasten the cap of the bottle.
2. Shake the bottle well to mix the oils completely.
3. Store the bottle in a dark and cool place.

Usage:

Shake the bottle well before use. Add a few drops of oil into your diffuser. Follow the manufacturer's instructions and use the diffuser as instructed.

Bye Bye Allergies

Ingredients:

- 15 drops peppermint oil
- 15 drops lavender oil
- 15 drops lemon oil

Method:

1. Add all the oils into a clean, dark dropper bottle. Fasten the cap of the bottle.
2. Shake the bottle well to mix the oils completely.
3. Store the bottle in a dark and cool place.

Usage:

Shake the bottle well before use. Add a few drops of oil into your diffuser. Follow the manufacturer's instructions and use the diffuser as instructed.

Bye Bye Insect Blend

Ingredients:

- 10 drops lemongrass oil
- 10 drops eucalyptus oil
- 10 drops thyme oil
- 10 drops basil oil

Method:

1. Add all the oils into a clean, dark dropper bottle. Fasten the cap of the bottle.
2. Shake the bottle well to mix the oils completely.
3. Store the bottle in a dark and cool place.

Usage:

Shake the bottle well before use. Add a few drops of oil into your diffuser. Follow the manufacturer's instructions and use the diffuser as instructed.

Repel the Bugs

Ingredients:

- 10 drops lemongrass oil
- 10 drops eucalyptus oil
- 10 drops thyme oil
- 10 drops rosemary oil
- 10 drops Melaleuca oil

Method:

1. Add all the oils into a clean, dark dropper bottle. Fasten the cap of the bottle.
2. Shake the bottle well to mix the oils completely.
3. Store the bottle in a dark and cool place.

Usage:

Shake the bottle well before use. Add a few drops of oil into your diffuser. Follow the manufacturer's instructions and use the diffuser as instructed.

Morning Sickness

Ingredients:

- 3-5 drops of peppermint oil or ginger oil or lemon oil or spearmint oil or lavender oil

Usage:

Shake the bottle well before use. Add a few drops of the chosen oil into your diffuser. You can also use any 2 of the above-mentioned oils. Follow the manufacturer's instructions and use the diffuser as instructed for 30 minutes every 4-6 hours.

Common Cold Relief Blend

Ingredients:

- 25 drops rosemary oil
- 20 drops peppermint oil
- 20 drops eucalyptus oil
- 10 drops lemon oil
- 15 drops cypress oil

Method:

1. Add all the oils into a clean, dark dropper bottle. Fasten the cap of the bottle.
2. Shake the bottle well to mix the oils completely.
3. Store the bottle in a dark and cool place.

Usage:

Shake the bottle well before use. Add a few drops of oil into your diffuser. Follow the manufacturer's instructions and use the diffuser as instructed.

Blend for Concentration

Ingredients:

- 30 drops lemon oil
- 30 drops rosemary oil
- 10 drops peppermint oil

Method:

1. Add all the oils into a clean, dark dropper bottle. Fasten the cap of the bottle.
2. Shake the bottle well to mix the oils completely.
3. Store the bottle in a dark and cool place.

Usage:

Shake the bottle well before use. Add a few drops of oil into your diffuser. Follow the manufacturer's instructions and use the diffuser as instructed.

To Combat Cold and Flu

Ingredients:

- 20 drops eucalyptus oil
- 20 drops peppermint oil
- 20 drops lavender oil
- 20 drops tea tree oil

Method:

1. Add eucalyptus oil and peppermint oil into a clean, dark dropper bottle. Fasten the cap of the bottle.
2. Add lavender oil and tea tree oil into another clean, dark dropper bottle. Fasten the cap of the bottle.
3. Shake the bottles well to mix the oils completely.
4. Store the bottles in a dark and cool place.

Usage:

Shake the bottle well before use.

Add 4 drops oil blend from each bottle into your diffuser (to combat daytime flu).

Add 4 drops oil from the lavender –tea tree blend into your diffuser (to combat nighttime flu)

Follow the manufacturer's instructions and use the diffuser as instructed.

Conclusion

Thank you once again for choosing this book.

I'm sure you are now itching to go on and try your own recipe blends and make the most of these essential oils. The fact is, nature has the answers for almost all problems, so it makes sense to go natural and use what is provided to us by Mother Nature in abundance.

These recipes will help you deal with a wide range of issues like stress, depression, allergies, snoring, sleeplessness, weight loss, cold, morning sickness etc. Rather than spending hundreds of dollars for store brought products, it makes a lot of sense to switch to your own essential oil recipes that you can use and reap benefits from.

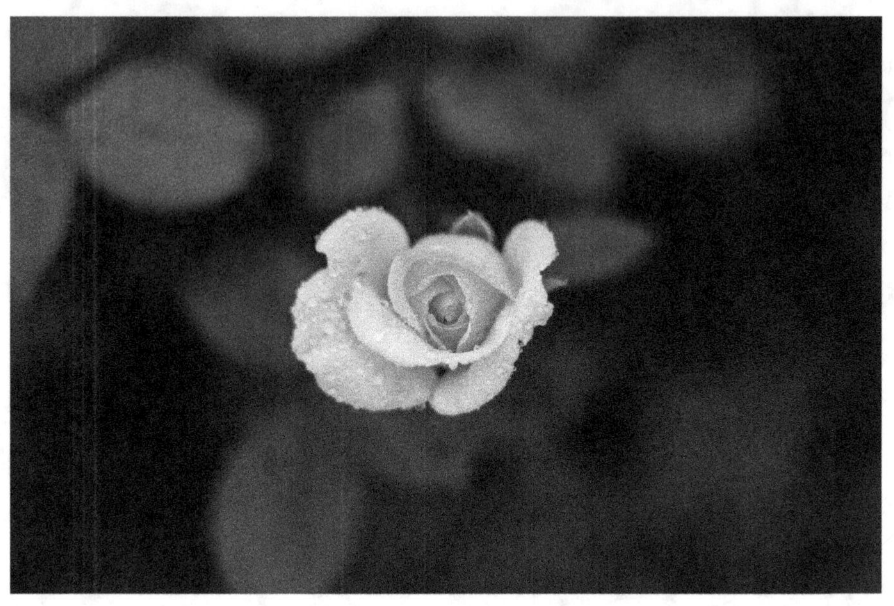

And finally, if you liked the book, I would like to ask you to do me the favor of leaving a review on Amazon.

Please go to your account on Amazon, or

paste in the link below.

http://amzn.to/2u6efd1

Thank you!